The Kidney Disease Solution

The Ultimate Kidney Disease Diet Cookbook

The Only Renal Diet Cookbook You Will Ever Need

By

Martha Stephenson

Copyright 2016 Martha Stephenson

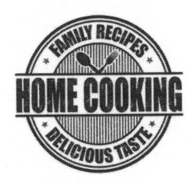

License Notes

No part of this Book can be reproduced in any form or by any means including print, electronic, scanning or photocopying unless prior permission is granted by the author.

All ideas, suggestions and guidelines mentioned here are written for informative purposes. While the author has taken every possible step to ensure accuracy, all readers are advised to follow information at their own risk. The author cannot be held responsible for personal and/or commercial damages in case of misinterpreting and misunderstanding any part of this Book

Table of Contents

Introduction

When you are first diagnosed with a disease, I know how difficult it can be to hear the news. However, when it comes to Kidney Disease the news doesn't have to be bad when you first hear it. The truth of the matter is that when you suffer from kidney disease, there are many lifestyle changes that you can make to help you manage your disease. One of the many changes you can make is to alter your diet and to eat kidney friendly meals.

That is exactly what you will find in this book. Inside of this book you will discover a few things about Kidney Disease such as what are the symptoms, what are the best types of food to eat to help manage your kidney disease as well as how kidney disease can be caused. You will also find over 25 delicious kidney friendly recipes that I know you are going to want to make as often as possible.

So, let's not waste any more time.

Let's get cooking!

What Is Kidney Disease?

In order to understand what kidney disease is we must first understand how your kidneys function normally. Inside of your body you have two kidneys that are about the size of your fist and are shaped like two small beans. When they are working properly you can eat healthy kidney friendly recipes to keep your entire body balanced by doing very important jobs that without them, would not be able to function normally. Some of the most important functions of your kidney include:

- Cleaning material waste from your bloodstream.
- Removing any excess water from your body.
- Helping to regulate your blood pressure to keep it within normal limits
- Helps to stimulate your bone marrow to make healthy red blood cells throughout your body.
- And help to control the amount of calcium and phosphorus with in your body at any given moment.

When you suffer from chronic kidney disease, your kidneys do not function properly and are unable to complete any of these important jobs that they need to do. While there is no cure at the moment for kidney failure, it is possible to live with chronic kidney disease and live a long and healthy life while helping your kidneys to function as best as they can.

What Are the Causes of Kidney Disease?

There is no set cause for kidney disease. Instead it is most often caused by variety of different things. Kidney disease can be most often caused by diabetes or high blood pressure, can afflict people of different races such as Hispanics, Native Americans and African-Americans, those with a greater risk of kidney failure, or those with kidney failure in their family.

Symptoms of Kidney Disease and Kidney Failure

Kidney failure is a very progressive disease which means that it does not happen overnight. There are many people who suffer from the early stages of kidney disease but do not show any symptoms. Symptoms usually occur in people during the later stages of kidney failure. Some of the symptoms of kidney disease can include:

- Nausea
- Having poor appetite
- Constant weakness
- Having trouble sleeping
- Increase tiredness
- Constant itching
- Increase weight loss, especially in the leg region
- Swelling around your feet and ankles
- Having low red blood cell count

The good news is that once you begin noticing the symptoms you can seek treatment. Once you seek treatment these symptoms will start to improve over time as well as your general health.

How The Kidney Diet Can Help Alleviate Kidney Disease?

Depending on what stage your kidney disease is currently at, your overall blood work results and the type of treatment you are seeking, the kidney diet can certainly help keep your kidneys healthy. While the diet itself may seem very overwhelming at first, the longer you follow it the easier it gets to get used to it and the healthier you will feel. In this section we will talk about some of the important components of the kidney diet so you can see how it will benefit you and your kidney disease in the long run.

Potassium

Potassium itself is a very important mineral that your body needs in order to thrive. It is also one of the important minerals that your body needs so that it can help balance out the amount of water between your cells and keep these levels at a normal level. Healthy kidneys help to remove any excess potassium that you have in your body through urination. However, when your kidneys are not functioning properly they cannot remove this excess potassium and it will build up in your blood.

While there are many different types of food that contain potassium it is important that you consume foods that are low in potassium rather than eating anything that has too much potassium.

Phosphorus

Phosphorus is another naturally occurring mineral that you can find in many foods today. Phosphorus helps to build strong and healthy bones but can damage your body if consumed in excess. Healthy kidneys are able to remove this extra phosphorus from your blood but if you suffer from kidney disease they are unable to do so. Once on the kidney diet you want to make sure that you consume foods that are low in phosphorus or do not contain any whatsoever. This means excluding such food items from your diet such as milk, nuts, dried beans, rice and beer.

Protein

Protein is one of the most important minerals that you can consume today. Not only is protein needed to repair tissue, but it also is needed to help build healthy muscle and help to prevent infection within your body. In order to stay healthy, you need to consume protein. On average you need to consume at least 40 to 65 grams of protein each day. However, if you are suffering from kidney disease you will need to reduce the amount of protein you take in by as much as only consuming up to 12% to 15% of your entire caloric intake per day.

Once following the kidney diet, you will not be consuming too much protein as this can prove too hard on your already malfunctioning kidneys. This may lead to you losing weight and having an increased risk of infection. However, it will help your kidneys out in the long run.

Fats

If you are the type of person that consumes too much fat on a daily basis, this is something that you are going to have to cut down on if you expect your kidneys to function normally. Not only consuming fat content increase your risk of heart disease, but it is also related to overall kidney disease as well. By following the kidney diet, you will be consuming fat sources but they will only be healthy fat sources such as olive oil or canola oil.

Sodium

While we all know that salt is something that we should not consume too much of, it is important to help regulate your body's normal water content and its normal blood pressure function. While normal kidneys can help filter out too much sodium from your body, with kidney disease it is not able to do so. That is why when following the kidney diet, you will reduce the amount of sodium that you take into your body.

Carbs and Fiber

Carbohydrates and fiber are important minerals that you need in order to protect your heart, your colon and healthy blood vessel function. While a diet high in fiber can help certainly reduce the risk of heart attack, when you suffer from kidney disease you are not getting enough fiber in your diet. This can lead to you suffering from diarrhea or constipation. When you follow the kidney diet, you will be increasing the amount of fiber that you take in which can help reduce the symptoms in the long run.

Fluid Intake

Depending on what stage of kidney disease you are suffering from you may need to limit the amount of fluids you take in on a daily basis. If you risk drinking too much liquid, you will risk suffering from fluid retention which can in turn lead to an increased blood pressure and swelling throughout your body.

Healthy Kidney Disease Diet Recipes

Kidney Friendly Deviled Eggs

This delicious and kidney friendly deviled eggs recipes makes deviled eggs that are on the sweet and tangy side. These are the perfect appetizers to serve to your friends and family without them realizing how beneficial they are for their body.

Makes: 6 Servings

Total Prep Time: 10 Minutes

Ingredients:

- 6 Eggs, Large in Size and Hardboiled
- 2 Tbsp. of Mayonnaise, Your Favorite Kind
- 1 tsp. of Vinegar, Cider Variety
- 1 tsp. of Sugar, White
- 1 tsp. of Mustard, Yellow in Color
- ½ tsp. of Onion, Powdered Variety
- Dash of Paprika, Optional

Directions:

1. The first thing that you will want to do is slice your eggs in half and remove the yolks from the inside. Place your egg yolks into a small sized bowl and set your whites aside.

2. Then mash your egg yolks finely using a fork until smooth and fluffy in consistency.

3. Add in your next 5 ingredients into your eggs yolks and mash thoroughly to evenly combine.

4. Stuff your egg whites with your egg yolk mixture until everything has been used up.

5. Season with a dash of paprika and enjoy whenever you are ready.

Easy Vegetable and Rice Skillet

If you are looking for a piping hot and delicious meal that will leave you feeling full for the entire day, then this is the perfect recipe for you. Filled with high quality and nutritious veggies and carbs, this is one dish that will help benefit your kidneys in the long run.

Makes: 3 Servings

Total Prep Time: 30 Minutes

Ingredients:

- 1 Onion, Medium in Size and Finely Chopped
- 1 Tbsp. of Butter, Unsalted Variety
- 2 Carrots, Medium in Size and Finely Sliced
- 2 Cups of Cauliflower, Cut into Florets
- 1 Cup of Rice, Uncooked
- 2 Cloves of Garlic, Minced
- 1 ½ Cups of Chicken Broth, Low in Sodium
- 1 Tbsp. of Parsley, Minced and Fresh
- ¼ tsp. of Pepper, For Taste

Directions:

1. The first thing that you will want to do is use a large sized skillet and place over medium heat. Once your skillet is hot enough add in your butter. Once fully melted add in your onions and cook until they are tender to the touch.

2. Then add in your carrots and continue to cook for an additional 5 minutes.

3. Add in your next 3 ingredients and stir thoroughly to combine. Cook for another minute.

4. Add in your broth and allow your mixture to come to a boil. Once your mixture is boiling, reduce the heat to low and cook for at least 20 to 25 minutes or until your rice is tender to the touch.

5. Remove from heat and season with y0ur parsley and pepper. Serve while still piping hot and enjoy.

Summer Time Antipasto Pasta Salad

This is a great tasting and healthy salad recipe that you can enjoy during the summer time months. Light and filling, this is a great dish to make if you want to impress your friends and family at your next summer gathering.

Makes: 8 Servings

Total Prep Time: 1 Hour

Ingredients:

- 16 Ounces of Pasta, Rotini Style and Fully Cooked
- ½ Pound of Chicken Breasts, Fully Cooked and Cut into Small Sized Cubed
- ¼ Pound of Parmesan Cheese, Freshly Grated
- 2 Peppers, Pepperoncini Variety
- 1/3 Cup of Basil, Fresh and Roughly Chopped
- 1 Cup of Vinegar, Red Wine Variety
- ¼ Cup of Olive Oil, Extra Virgin Variety and Basil Flavored
- ½ Cup of Olive Oil, Extra Virgin Variety and Garlic Flavored
- ¼ Cup of Olive Oil, Extra Virgin Variety and Plain
- ¼ tsp. of Black Pepper, For Taste

Directions:

1. Toss all of your ingredients into a large sized bowl and toss thoroughly to mix.

2. Place into your fridge to chill for the next hour.

3. Remove from fridge and toss again. Serve whenever you are ready.

Kidney Friendly Chicken Fajitas

Who isn't a huge fan of fajitas? Well, if you love authentic fajitas then I know you are definitely going to love this recipe. Easy to make and easy on your kidneys, feel free to make this dish any time of the week.

Makes: 8 Servings

Total Prep Time: 30 Minutes

Ingredients:

- 6 Chicken Thighs, Boneless, Skinless and Cut into Thin Strips
- 1 Onion, Large in Size, Yellow in Color and Sliced Thinly
- 1 Red Pepper, Large in Size, Cored and Sliced Thinly
- 1 to 2 Tbsp. of Chili, Powdered Variety
- ½ to 1 Tbsp. of Cumin, Ground
- Dash of Black Pepper, For Taste
- Dash of Cilantro, Fresh, Roughly Chopped and for Garnish
- 8 Tortillas, Floured Variety
- Dash of Olive Oil, Extra Virgin Variety

Directions:

1. The first thing that you will want to do is use a large sized skillet and heat up your olive oil over medium heat.

2. Once your oil is hot enough add in your peppers and cook for at least 5 to 6 minutes or until tender to the touch. Once tender add in your onions and continue to cook until your onions are tender to the touch. Once tender remove your peppers and onions from the skillet and set aside for later use.

3. Then add your chicken to your skillet with some more oil and cook for the next 8 to 10 minutes.

4. After this time add in your onions and peppers and cook until completely heated through.

5. Season with a touch of your seasoning and stir thoroughly to coat.

6. Remove from heat and garnish with your cilantro. Serve with your tortillas and enjoy whenever you are ready. Enjoy.

Kidney Friendly Coleslaw

If you have a family picnic or barbecue coming up, then this is one dish that I know you are going to want to make. Easy to put together and incredibly nutritious, your entire family will be begging you for the recipe.

Makes: 4 to 5 Servings

Total Prep Time: 1 Hour

Ingredients:

- 3 to 4 Cups of Cabbage, Finely Shredded
- 3 Carrots, Baby Variety and Finely Shredded
- ¼ tsp. of Pepper, For Taste
- ¼ tsp. of Fennel, Ground
- 3 Tbsp. of Vinegar, Rice Variety
- 3 Tbsp. of Mayonnaise, Your Favorite Kind
- 1 ½ Packs of Sweet and Low

Directions:

1. The first thing that you will want to do is mix all of your ingredients in a large sized bowl and toss to thoroughly combine.

2. Cover and place in your fridge to chill for at least 1 hour.

3. After this time serve your dish whenever you are ready. Enjoy.

Easy Chicken Salad

This healthy chicken salad recipe is packed with nutritious green onions, fennel and celery, making it the ultimate salad recipe for you to enjoy. For the tastiest results I highly recommend serving this dish on a bed of lettuce or in a sandwich. Either way I know you will enjoy it.

Makes: 3 Servings

Total Prep Time: 1 Hour

Ingredients:

- 1 Cup of Chicken, Fully Cooked and Finely Chopped
- ¼ Cup of Celery, Fresh and Finely Chopped
- 2 Tbsp. of Green Onions, Finely Sliced
- 3 Tbsp. of Mayonnaise, Your Favorite Kind
- 1 tsp. of Pickles, Sweet Variety and Finely Chopped
- 1/8 tsp. of Fennel, Ground
- ¼ tsp. of Garlic, Ground
- ¼ tsp. of Salt, For Taste and Optional
- ¼ tsp. of Black Pepper, For Taste

Directions:

1. The first thing that you will want to do is mix all of your ingredients together in a large sized bowl until thoroughly mixed together.

2. Cover with some plastic wrap and place into your fridge to chill for the next hour.

3. After this time remove from fridge and serve whenever you are ready.

Healthy Cauliflower Soup

If you are looking for the ultimate nutritious soup recipe to enjoy, then this is the perfect soup recipe for you to make. Packed full of healthy cauliflower, celery and carrots, this is one dish that is not only healthy for your kidneys, but healthy for your entire body as well.

Makes: 4 Servings

Total Prep Time: 25 Minutes

Ingredients:

- 3 Cups of Water, Warm
- 1 Cup of Cauliflower, Frozen, Thawed and Finely Chopped
- ¼ of a Cube of Bouillon, Chicken Variety and Low in Sodium
- ½ of an Onion, Medium in Size and Finely Chopped
- ¼ Cup of Celery, Fresh and Finely Chopped
- 3 Carrots, Baby Variety and Finely Sliced
- 1/8 tsp. of Basil, Dried and Roughly Chopped
- 1 Tbsp. of Mayonnaise, Your Favorite Kind
- 3 Tbsp. of Cream Cheese, Soft
- 1 Tbsp. of Margarine
- ½ tsp. of Salt, For Taste
- ¼ tsp. of Pepper, For Taste
- 1/3 tsp. of Garlic, Granulated Variety

- 1 Tbsp. of Flour, For Thickening
- 1 Tbsp. of Butter, For Thickening

Directions:

1. Use a large sized soup pot and place in your first 6 ingredients into it. Stir to combine and heat over high heat to bring to a boil.

2. Once your mixture is boiling reduce the heat to low and continue to cook until your veggies are tender to the touch.

3. Add in your remaining ingredients except for your last two ingredients. Stir to thoroughly combine and continue to cook for another 3 to 5 minutes.

5. Add in your next 2 ingredients and continue to cook until your soup is thick in consistency.

6. Remove from heat and serve whenever you are ready. Enjoy!

Nutritious Asparagus and Chicken Linguini

This delicious asparagus and chicken linguini recipe incorporates different Italian classic ingredients such as white wine, garlic, parmesan cheese and olive oil, making this the perfect kidney friendly dish to enjoy when you are craving Italian.

Makes: 4 Servings

Total Prep Time: 25 Minutes

Ingredients:

- 6 Ounces of Linguine, Fully Cooked
- 1 Onion, Small in Size and Finely Chopped
- 2 Cloves of Garlic, Minced
- 1 Tbsp. of Olive Oil, Extra Virgin Variety
- 2 tsp. of Butter, Unsalted Variety
- ½ Pound of Asparagus, Fresh, Trimmed and Cut into Small Pieces
- ½ Pound of Chicken Breasts, Fully Cooked and Cut into Small Cubes
- 2 Tbsp. of Wine, White in Color and Your Favorite Kind
- 2 Tbsp. of Parmesan Cheese, Finely Shredded
- 1 Tbsp. of Lemon Juice, Fresh
- 1/8 tsp. of Pepper, For Taste

Directions:

1. The first thing that you will want to do is cook your linguine according to the directions on the package. Once cooked drain and set aside for later use.

2. Then use a medium sized skillet placed over medium heat. Add your oil and once the oil is hot enough add in your garlic and butter and cook until your garlic is tender.

3. Next add in your asparagus and fully cooked chicken. Cook for the next 2 minutes.

4. Then add in your wine and continue to cook for the next 2 minutes or until your liquid is reduced by at least half.

5. Toss your linguine into your skillet and remove from heat. Toss until everything is mixed together.

6. Serve with a garnishing of more parmesan cheese and serve while still piping hot. Enjoy.

Creamy Style Chicken Mac and Cheese

If you are a huge fan of mac and cheese, then this is one dish you are going to fall in love with. Made with wholesome chicken, cream mac and cheese and creamy mayonnaise, making it a delicious dish you will want to enjoy over and over again.

Makes: 4 Servings

Total Prep Time: 20 Minutes

Ingredients:

- 4 Ounces of Chicken Breast, Fully Cooked and Cut into Small Cubes
- 2 Tbsp. of Margarine, Soft
- 2 Tbsp. of Flour, All Purpose Variety
- 1 ½ Cup of Water, Warm
- ¼ of a Cube of Bouillon, Chicken Variety and Low in Sodium
- 2 Tbsp. of Cream Cheese, Soft
- 1 Tbsp. of Mayonnaise, Your Favorite Kind
- ½ tsp. of Onion, Powdered Variety
- ¼ tsp. of Black Pepper, For Taste
- ¼ tsp. of Salt, For Taste
- ¼ tsp. of Garlic, Powdered Variety

- 3 Cups of Macaroni, Elbow Variety and Fully Cooked
- 1 tsp. of Lemon Juice, Fresh and Optional

Directions:

1. The first thing that you will want to do is add your margarine and flour together into a large sized skillet. Place over medium heat and cook for a few minutes, making sure to whisk thoroughly to prevent any lumps from forming.

2. Next dissolve your bouillon in some water and add it to your skillet, whisking thoroughly until your mixture is thick in consistency.

3. Add in your cream cheese and mayonnaise and allow to melt completely.

4. Whisk in your remaining ingredients and toss thoroughly to coat.

5. Remove from heat and serve whenever you are ready. Enjoy!

Cranberry and Lemon Muffins

These delicious muffins are a great treat to make for yourself if you have a sweet tooth that needs to be satisfied. Made with delicious and nutritious cranberries and packed full of lemon zest, I guarantee even the pickiest of eaters are going to love it.

Makes: 24 Muffins

Total Prep Time: 40 Minutes

Ingredients:

- ¾ Cup of Butter, Unsalted Variety and Warmed to Room Temperature
- 1 ½ Cup of Sugar, White
- 3 Eggs, Large in Size and Beaten
- 1 ½ tsp. of Vanilla, Pure
- 1 Cup of Sour Cream, Soft
- ¼ Cup of Lemon Juice, Fresh
- 1 Tbsp. of Lemon, Zest Only
- 2 ½ Cups of Flour, All Purpose Variety
- 2 tsp. of Baker's Style of Baking Powder
- ½ tsp. of Baker's Style Baking Soda
- ¾ Cup of Cranberries, Sweetened Variety and Dried

Directions:

1. The first thing that you will want to do is preheat an oven to 350 degrees. While your oven is heating up grease a muffin pan with a generous amount of cooking spray.

2. Then use a large sized bowl and cream your butter and sugar together using an electric mixer until fluffy in consistency. This should take at least 4 minutes.

3. Then add in your eggs, making sure to add them in one at a time along with your next 4 ingredients.

4. Using another large sized bowl mix together your next 3 ingredients until thoroughly combined. Mix in with your butter mixture until a batter begins to form.

5. Gently fold in your cranberries until evenly incorporated.

6. Pour your batter generously into your muffin pans.

7. Place into your oven to bake for the next 25 to 30 minutes or until your muffins are light brown in color.

8. After this time remove your muffins and allow to cool before serving.

No Sugar Chocolate Chip Cookies

If you are looking for a way to satisfy your strongest sweet tooth, then this is the perfect dessert recipe for you. With no sugar added into these cookies, you will never be able to taste the difference.

Makes: 18 Servings

Total Prep Time: 20 Minutes

Ingredients:

- 1 Cup of Flour, All Purpose Variety
- ½ tsp. of Baker's Style Baking Soda
- ¼ tsp. of Salt, For Taste
- ½ Cup of Margarine, Soft
- 4 tsp. of Liquid Sugar, Substitute Variety
- ½ tsp. of Vanilla, Pure
- 1 Egg, Large in Size and Beaten
- ½ Cup of Chocolate Chips, Semi-Sweet Variety

Directions:

1. The first thing that you will want to do is preheat your oven to 250 degrees.

2. While your oven is heating up use a large sized mixing bowl and sift together all of your dry ingredients until they are thoroughly combine.

3. Then cream together your margarine and next 3 ingredients in another mixing bowl until evenly mixed and crumbly.

4. Add your margarine ingredients to your flour mixture and stir well to evenly combine.

5. Gently fold in your chocolate chips.

6. Drop by the tablespoon onto a lightly greased baking sheet.

7. Place into your oven to bake for the next 10 minutes or until completely cooked through.

8. Remove from your oven and allow to cool slightly before serving. Enjoy.

Easy Berry and Cherry Pie

If you are looking for a delicious dessert dish to serve to your entire family, then this is the perfect dish for you to make. It is incredibly easy to make when you use a ready-made pie, making it a dessert dish that can be ready to satisfy your entire family in a matter of minutes.

Makes: 8 Servings

Total Prep Time: 45 Minutes

Ingredients:

- 1 Cup of Cherries, Canned Variety, Unsweetened, drained with Juice Reserved
- 1 Cup of Raspberries, Canned Variety, Unsweetened, drained with Juice Reserved
- ¾ Cup of Raspberry and Cheery Juices, with Water Added if Needed
- 1 Tbsp. of Cornstarch
- ¼ of Almond, Extract
- 2 Pie Crusts, Pre-made

Directions:

1. Using a small sized saucepan and combine both of your juices, sugar and cornstarch together. Cook over low heat until your mixture is thick in consistency, making sure to stir often.

2. Then add in your cherries, almond extract and raspberries and stir until thoroughly combined.

3. Place your pie crust into your pie pan. Pour your cherry mixture into it and cover with your second pie crust, making sure to seal the edges nicely. Cut small slits into the top of your crust.

4. Preheat your oven to 450 degrees. Once your oven is hot enough add your pie into your oven for the next 15 minutes.

5. After this time reduce the heat in your oven to 375 degrees and continue to bake your pie for the next 25 to 30 minutes or until your crust is golden brown in color.

6. Remove from your oven and allow to cool slightly before serving.

Vegan Style Pizza

If you are looking for a healthy vegetarian or vegan friendly dish, then this is the perfect late night dinner meal to make. This pizza dish is made using homemade pizza dough, roasted onions and garlic, making this a dish you will fall in love with.

Makes: 12 Servings

Total Prep Time: 1 Hour and 10 Minutes

Ingredients for Your Pizza Dough:

- ¼ Cup of Water, Warm
- 1 Pack of Dry Yeast, Active
- 2 Tbsp. of Sugar, White
- 2 Tbsp. of Oil, Canola Variety
- 1 ½ Cup of Milk, Rice Variety and Warm
- 3 to 4 Cups of Flour, All Purpose Variety

Ingredients for Your Toppings:

- 2 Heads of Garlic
- 5 Onions, Red in Color and Thinly Sliced
- Some Rosemary, Dried and Roughly Chopped
- Some Cooking Spray

Directions:

1. The first thing that you will want to do is prepare your pizza dough.

2. While your oven is heating up, mix together your yeast and warm water and allow to sit for the next 5 minutes.

3. Then take a large sized mixing bowl and combine all of your dough ingredients together. Stir well to evenly combine. Knead for the next 5 to 10 minutes.

4. Spray a separate mixing bowl with a generous amount of cooking spray and place your kneaded dough into it. Cover with some plastic wrap and allow to rise in a warm place for the next 30 minutes.

5. After this time punch your dough down and divide it to 6 even sized pieces. Roll out these pieces into small sized bowls. Set aside.

6. Next preheat your oven to 450 degrees. While your oven is heating up peel your garlic and place the cloves in some aluminum foil. Spray the garlic with cooking spray and seal the foil.

7. Place into your oven to roast for the next 30 to 40 minutes or until tender to the touch.

8. Next peel and finely slice your onions. Place onto a generously greased baking sheet and place into your oven to roast for the next 30 to 40 minutes, making sure to turn them every 15 minutes.

9. Once roasted place your garlic cloves and onions onto your rolled out dough. Top with your herbs.

10. Place into your oven to bake for the next 12 to 15 minutes or until your crust is light brown in color.

11. Remove from oven and allow to cool slightly before serving.

Sweet Tasting Apple Cake with Honey Sauce

Here is yet another sweet tasting dessert dish that I know you and your entire family are going to fall in love with. This cake is made using fresh lemon juice and spiced with nutmeg, making this the perfect dish to enjoy during the holiday seasoning.

Makes: 9 Servings

Total Prep Time: 1 Hour and 10 Minutes

Ingredients:

- 1/3 Cup of Lemon Juice, Fresh
- 3 Cups of Apples, Peeled and Finely Diced
- 3 Tbsp. of Margarine, Fresh
- ½ Cup of Sugar, White
- ½ Cup of Honey, Raw
- 1 Egg, Large in Size and Beaten
- 2 Cups of Flour, All Purpose Variety
- 1 tsp. of Baker's Style Baking Powder
- ½ tsp. of Baker's Style Baking Soda
- ¼ tsp. of Nutmeg, Ground
- 2 ½ tsp. of Cornstarch
- ½ Cup of Honey, Raw
- 1/3 Cup of Water, Warm
- 1 Tbsp. of Lemon Peel, Freshly Grated

- 3 Tbsp. of Lemon Juice, Fresh
- 1 Tbsp. of Margarine, Soft
- Dash of Nutmeg, Ground

Directions:

1. The first thing that you will want to do is preheat your oven to 350 degrees.

2. While your oven is heating up pour your first lemon juice over the top of your apples and toss thoroughly to coat. Set aside for later use.

3. Then cream together your margarine and sugar together in a medium sized bowl until thoroughly combined. Add in your honey and use an electric mixer to beat well. Add in your egg and mix again.

4. Using another bowl add in your next 4 ingredients and stir to combine. Add to your margarine mixture. Add in your apples and stir again to coat.

5. Pour your apple mixture into a generously greased baking dish and place into your oven to bake for the next hour.

6. While your apple mixture is cooking, make your sauce. To do this mix together your cornstarch, water and honey together in a small sized saucepan place over medium heat.

7. Add in your lemon peel and continue to cook for the next 5 minutes or until thick in consistency, making sure to stir occasionally.

8. Remove from heat and add in your remaining ingredients until thoroughly combined.

9. Remove your cake from your oven and allow to cool completely before pouring your sauce over the top. Serve whenever you are ready.

Filling Shrimp Scampi Linguine

If you are a huge fan of traditional Italian cuisine, then this is a tasty dish I know you are going to fall in love with. This dish is toss with delicious shrimp, olive oil, roasted garlic, white wine and served on top of a bed of linguine.

Makes: 4 Servings

Total Prep Time: 25 Minutes

Ingredients:

- 1 Tbsp. of Olive Oil, Extra Virgin Variety
- 1 Clove of Garlic, Minced
- ½ Pound of Shrimp, Peeled and Deveined
- ¼ Cup of White Wine, Dry and Your Favorite Kind
- 1 Tbsp. of Lemon Juice, Fresh
- ½ tsp. of Basil, Dried
- 1 Tbsp. of Parsley, Fresh and Roughly Chopped
- 4 Ounces of Linguine, Uncooked

Directions:

1. First heat up your oil in a large sized skillet placed over medium heat. Once your oil is hot enough add in your garlic and shrimp.

2. Cook until your shrimp turns pink in color.

3. Then add in your next 4 ingredients and continue to cook for the next 5 minutes.

4. While your shrimp mixture is cooking cook your linguine in a pot of boiling water seasoned with salt until your linguine is tender to the touch. Once tender, drain and serve.

5. Top your linguine with your shrimp mixture and serve while piping hot. Enjoy.

Hearty Onion Steak

This is a great tasting dish packed full of nutritious ingredients that your kidneys need while suffering from kidney disease. This dish is slowly simmer to make a dish that you will never be able to get enough of.

Makes: 8 Servings

Total Prep Time: 1 Hour and 15 Minutes

Ingredients:

- ¼ Cup of Flour, All Purpose Variety
- 1/8 tsp. of Pepper, For Taste
- 1 ½ Pound of Round Steak, At Least ¾ of an Inch Thick
- 2 Tbsp. of Oil, Olive Variety
- 1 Cup of Water, Warm
- 1 Clove of Garlic, Minced
- 1 Bay Leaf, Dried
- ¼ tsp. of Thyme, Dried and Crushed
- 3 Onions, Medium in Size and Finely Sliced

Directions:

1. The first thing that you will want to do is cut your steak into 8 equaled sized pieces.

2. Then combine your flour and pepper together in a small sized bowl until thoroughly combined. Add to your meat and pound it with a tenderizer.

3. Next heat up your oil in a large sized skillet, cook your meat and browning it thoroughly on all sides. Once brown in color remove from your skillet and set aside for later use.

4. Next combine your next 5 ingredients together and add to your skillet. Bring this mixture to a boil.

5. Add your meat back into this mixture and add in your onions. Cover and allow to simmer for the next hour.

6. After this time remove from heat and serve while still piping hot. Enjoy.

Light Chicken Tarragon

This light dish is smothered in stroganoff style cream sauce and serve over a bed of hot noodles, making it the perfect dish to make if you are looking for something hearty yet filling.

Makes: 12 Servings

Total Prep Time: 30 Minutes

Ingredients:

- 8 Chicken Breasts, Cut into Halves, Boneless and Skinless Variety
- 2 Tbsp. of Margarine, Soft
- 2 Cups of Mushrooms, Fresh and Cut into Halves
- 2 Cloves of Garlic, Minced
- 3 Tbsp. of Sherry, Dried
- ½ tsp. of Tarragon, Dried and Crushed
- ½ tsp. of Lemon and Pepper Seasoning
- 1 ¾ Cups of Chicken Broth, Sodium Free and Homemade Preferable
- 1/3 Cup of Flour, All Purpose Variety
- ¼ Cup of Sour Cream, Your Favorite Kind
- Some Noodles, Egg Variety and Fully Cooked

Directions:

1. The first thing that you will want to do is melt your margarine in a large sized skillet placed over medium heat.

2. Once your margarine is fully melted add in your first 6 ingredients. Toss to combine and cook for the next 10 to 12 minutes or until your chicken is fully cooked through. Make sure that you turn your chicken at least once.

3. Then remove your chicken and mushrooms from your skillet and place into a bag with your broth and flour. Shake well until thoroughly coated.

4. Add this mixture back into your skillet and cook over medium to high heat until it begins to bubble.

5. After this time remove at least half a cup of your broth from the skillet and add in your sour cream.

6. Continue to cook until completely heated through before removing from heat.

7. Serve your dish over a bed of hot noodles and serve while still piping hot.

Classic Meatloaf

If you are a huge fan of meatloaf, then I know you are going to love making this kidney friendly dish for yourself. Made with savory mushrooms, light brown sugar, roasted onions and topped with cheese, this is one meatloaf dish you are going to want to enjoy over and over again.

Makes: 8 Servings

Total Prep Time: 1 Hour and 5 Minutes

Ingredients for Your Loaf:

- 2 Eggs, Large in Size and Beaten
- ¾ Cup of Milk, Whole
- 2/3 Cup of Bread Crumbs, Dried
- 2 Tbsp. of Onions, Finely Diced
- ½ tsp. of Sage, Dried
- 1 ½ Pound of Beef, Lean and Ground
- ½ Cup of Mushrooms, Fresh and Finely Sliced

Ingredients for Your Topping:

- ¼ Cup of Ketchup, Sodium Free
- 2 Tbsp. of Brown Sugar, Light and Packed
- 1 tsp. of Mustard, Dried
- ¼ tsp. of Nutmeg, Ground
- ¼ Cup of Cheddar Cheese, Finely Shredded

Directions:

1. The first thing that you will want to do is preheat your oven to 350 degrees.

2. While your oven is heating up mix together all of your ingredients for your loaf together until evenly mixed. Pat this mixture into a large sized generously greased loaf pan.

3. Place into your oven to bake for the next hour. After this time remove from your oven.

4. Then mix together all of your ingredients for your topping in a medium sized bowl until evenly combined. Pour this mixture over your loaf and top off with your shredded cheese.

5. Return your pan back into your oven to bake just until your cheese fully melts.

6. Remove and allow to cool slightly before serving. Enjoy.

Herb Smothered Fish

If you are a huge fan of traditional fish recipes, then this is one fish recipe I know you are going to want to make over and over again. This fish dish incorporates delicious fish fillets baked to perfect with spices and a cream Parmesan topping.

Makes: 8 Servings

Total Prep Time: 25 Minutes

Ingredients:

- 8 1 ½ inch Thick Salmon Fillets,
- ½ Cup of Mayonnaise, Your Favorite Kind
- ½ Cup of Sour Cream
- ¼ Cup of Parmesan Cheese, Freshly Grated
- 4 Tbsp. of Chives, Freshly Chopped
- 2 Tbsp. of Parsley, Fresh and Roughly Chopped
- ½ tsp. of Onion, Powdered Variety
- ½ tsp. of Dill, Dried
- ½ tsp. of Mustard, Dried
- Dash of Black Pepper, For Taste

Directions:

1. The first thing that you will want to do is preheat your oven to 350 degrees.

2. Then place your salmon fillets into a shallow pan greased with margarine.

3. Then blend the rest of your ingredients together in a blend until evenly mixed. Spread this mixture on top of your salmon fillet.

4. Place into your oven to bake for the next 20 minutes or until your fillets are easily flaked off with a fork.

5. Remove from oven and serve immediately. Enjoy.

Delicious Grilled Sesame Style Chicken Breasts

This is another great tasting chicken recipe to make if you are looking to enjoy a tasty and savory dinner dish. This chicken dish is smothered in savory honey and ginger glaze that you will want to make over and over again.

Makes: 4 Servings

Total Prep Time: 20 Minutes

Ingredients:

- 1 Tbsp. of Sesame Seeds, Lightly Toasted
- 2 tsp. of Ginger, Freshly Grated
- 2 Tbsp. of Honey, Raw
- 1 Tbsp. of Soy Sauce, Low in Sodium
- 1 Tbsp. of Sherry, Cooking Variety
- Some Cooking Spray
- 1, 4 Ounce Chicken Breast, Skinless and Cut into Halves

Directions:

1. The first thing that you will want to do is combine your first 5 ingredients together in a small sized bowl until evenly mixed. Set aside for later use.

2. Then use a mallet and pound your chicken breast until it is a ¼ of an inch thick.

3. Next spray a grill with a generous amount of cooking spray.

4. Once your grill is preheated place your chicken onto it and cook until completely done, making sure to baste it with your soy sauce mixture ever couple of minutes.

5. Remove from grill and serve whenever you are ready.

Classic French Onion Soup

If you are looking for an easy and classic dish to make, you can't go wrong with making this dish for your soup. This classic soup dish is made using tasty cognac with low sodium croutons, making it the perfect dish to help your kidneys function while satisfying your taste buds at the same time.

Makes: 4 Servings

Total Prep Time: 30 Minutes

Ingredients:

- 4 Onions, Large in Size, Red in Color and Finely Sliced
- 1 Tbsp. of Butter, Soft
- 2 Tbsp. of Cognac
- 4 Cups of Vegetable Stock, Roasted and Homemade Preferable
- 4 Croutons, Large in Size and Low in Sodium

Directions:

1. The first thing that you will want to do is melt your butter in a large sized soup pot.

2. Once your butter is melted add in your onions and cook over medium heat until they are tender to the touch, making sure to stir it occasionally. This should take at least 15 minutes.

3. Next add in your stock and bring your mixture to a simmer. Allow your mixture to simmer over low heat for the next 15 minutes.

4. Serve with your low sodium croutons and enjoy while still piping hot.

Cajun Style Pork Chops

If you are looking for a dish that will add a bit of spice to your life, then this is the perfect recipe for you to make. Made with spicy herbs and hot sauce, you can't go wrong with this recipe.

Makes: 4 Hours

Total Prep Time: 40 Minutes

Ingredients:

- ¼ tsp. of Paprika
- ¼ tsp. of Garlic, Powdered Variety
- ¼ tsp. of Thyme, Dried
- ¼ tsp. of Mustard, Dry
- ¼ tsp. of Sage, Ground
- ¼ tsp. of Cumin, Ground
- 1/8 tsp. of Pepper, For Taste
- 4, 4 Ounce Pork Chops, At Least ½ Inch in Thickness
- 1 Onion, Small in Size and Finely Sliced
- 1 Tbsp. of Margarine, Soft
- 1 tsp. of Parsley Flakes, Dried
- 1/8 tsp. of Garlic, Powdered Variety
- 2 to 3 Drops of Hot Sauce, Your Favorite Kind

Directions:

1. The first thing that you will want to do is combine your first 7 ingredients together on some wax paper until thoroughly mixed together.

2. Then coat your pork chops on both sides in this mixture and place into a large sized baking dish.

3. Top each of your pork chops with your onions and cover with some wax paper.

4. Place into your microwave for the next 5 minutes, making sure to rotate. Then continue to microwave for the next 25 to 30 minutes, making sure to rotate every 5 minutes. Continue to cook until tender.

5. Next combine your remaining ingredients together in a small sized bowl and pour over your pork chops.

6. Continue to microwave until your pork chops are thoroughly cooked through.

7. Remove from your microwave and serve whenever you are ready. Enjoy.

Traditional Chile Verde

This is a traditional Mexican style stew that I know you are going to want to enjoy over and over again. For the tastiest results serve this dish with your favorite kind of tortillas to make it a filling dish you won't want to resist.

Makes: 5 Servings

Total Prep Time: 25 Minutes

Ingredients:

- 1 Pound of Pork, Cut into Small Chunks
- 1 Potato, Medium in size and Finely Diced
- 1 Onion, Finely Chopped
- 1 to 2 Cups of Water, Warm
- ½ Cup of Green Chile, Finely Chopped
- ½ tsp. of Garlic, Powdered Variety
- ½ tsp. of Salt, For Taste
- ½ tsp. of Black Pepper, For Taste
- Some Tortillas, Your Favorite Kind and for Serving
- Dash of Red Chiles, Powdered Variety and Optional

Directions:

1. The first thing that you will want to do is brown your pork thoroughly on all sides with your potatoes in a large sized skillet placed over medium heat.

2. Then add in your onions and continue to cook until tender to the touch.

3. Add in your remaining ingredients and reduce your heat to low. Allow to simmer until your water has completely evaporated and until your ingredients are tender to the touch.

4. Remove from heat and serve your dish with your favorite tortillas. Enjoy.

Filling Meatball Soup

If you are a huge fan of meatballs, then this is one delicious soup recipe I know you are going to want to enjoy every day of the week. This dish is made using fresh ground beef, spicy jalapenos and fresh tomatoes, making this a dish you won't be able to resist.

Makes: 12 Servings

Total Prep Time: 50 Minutes

Ingredients:

- 1 ½ Pounds of Beef, Lean and Ground
- ½ tsp. of Garlic, Salted Variety
- 1 tsp. of Cumin, Ground
- 1 Cup of White Tice, Uncooked
- 6 Cups of Water, Warm
- 1 Tomato, Medium in Size and Finely Chopped
- 1 Cup of Onion, Finely Chopped
- 1 Tbsp. of Jalapeno, Finely Chopped

Directions:

1. The first thing that you will want to do is season your beef with your garlic salt and ground cumin. Season well until your beef is thoroughly coated

2. Add in your rice and form your mixture into 24 even sized meatballs.

3. Place your meatballs into a large sized pot and add enough water to cover them.

4. Bring your dish to a simmer over low heat and then add in your next 3 ingredients.

5. Cover and continue to cook for the next 45 minutes.

6. After this time remove and serve whenever you are ready.

Hearty Beef Soup

Here is yet another great tasting soup recipe you are going to want to make during the cold winter months. It will leave you feeling full and satisfied.

Makes: 8 Servings

Total Prep Time: 35 Minutes

Ingredients:

- 1 ½ Pounds of Beef Chuck
- 1 Green Chile, Sliced into Rings
- 2 Potatoes, Medium in Size and Diced Finely
- ¼ Cup of Onion, Finely Chopped
- 1 Clove of Garlic, Minced
- ¼ tsp. of Salt, For Taste
- ½ Cup of Tomato, Finely Chopped
- 2 Cups of Water, Warm

Directions:

1. The first thing that you will want to do is cut your beef into small sized cubes.

2. Then use a large sized skillet and set over medium heat. Add in your oil and once it is hot enough fry your potatoes until tender to the touch.

3. Next add in your beef and cook until brown in color.

4. Add in your next 4 ingredients. Cook for the next 4 minutes until soft to the touch.

5. Add your water and cover. Cook for the next 10 minutes before removing from heat.

6. Serve with tortillas while still piping hot. Enjoy.

Conclusion

There you have it!

I hope that by the end of this book you have learned more about kidney disease such as what are the usual symptoms associated with it, how it can occur and what types of food you should eat to help boost your kidney's performance while still suffering from this disease. I also hope that you have found the 25 different kidney friendly recipes you have found in this book to be especially helpful in helping you manage your disease so you can get back to living a healthier and happier lifestyle.

So, what is the next step for you?

The next step for you to take is to begin managing your disease through the use of this healthy diet and by making all of the recipes you have found in this book. Once you have accomplished that then you should begin finding other kidney friendly recipes and begin making them as well.

Good luck!

About the Author

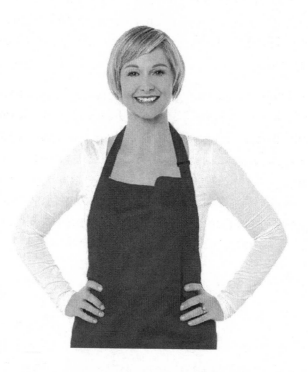

Martha is a chef and a cookbook author. She has had a love of all things culinary since she was old enough to help in the kitchen, and hasn't wanted to leave the kitchen since. She was born and raised in Illinois, and grew up on a farm, where she acquired her love for fresh, delicious foods. She learned many of her culinary abilities from her mother; most importantly, the need to cook with fresh, homegrown ingredients if at all possible, and how to create an amazing recipe that everyone wants. This gave her the perfect way to share her skill with the world; writing cookbooks to spread the message that fresh, healthy food really can, and does, taste delicious. Now that she is a mother, it is more important than ever to make sure that healthy food is available to the next generation. She hopes to become a household name in cookbooks for her delicious recipes, and healthy outlook.

Martha is now living in California with her high school sweetheart, and now husband, John, as well as their infant daughter Isabel, and two dogs; Daisy and Sandy. She is a stay at home mom, who is very much looking forward to expanding their family in the next few years to give their daughter some siblings. She enjoys cooking with, and for, her family and friends, and is waiting impatiently for the day she can start cooking with her daughter.

For a complete list of my published books, please, visit my Author's Page...

https://www.amazon.com/author/martha-stephenson

Author's Afterthoughts

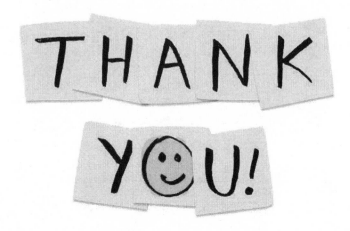

Thanks ever so much to each of my cherished readers for investing the time to read this book!

I know you could have picked from many other books but you chose this one. So a big thanks for downloading this book and reading all the way to the end.

If you enjoyed this book or received value from it, I'd like to ask you for a favor. Please take a few minutes to post an honest and heartfelt review on Amazon.com. Your support does make a difference and helps to benefit other people.

Thanks!

Martha Stephenson

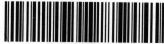

Made in the USA
Charleston, SC
07 June 2016